STARK LIBRARY

NOV 2020

HEALTH CARE CAREERS IN 2 YEARS™

JUMP-STARTING A CAREER IN RADIOLOGY

JASON PORTERFIELD

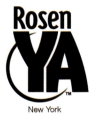

New York

Published in 2019 by The Rosen Publishing Group, Inc.
29 East 21st Street, New York, NY 10010

Copyright © 2019 by The Rosen Publishing Group, Inc.

First Edition

All rights reserved. No part of this book may be reproduced in any form without permission in writing from the publisher, except by a reviewer.

Library of Congress Cataloging-in-Publication Data

Names: Porterfield, Jason, author.
Title: Jump-starting a career in radiology / Jason Porterfield.
Description: First edition. | New York: Rosen YA, 2019. | Series: Health care careers in 2 years | Audience: Grades 7–12. | Includes bibliographical references and index.
Identifiers: LCCN 2018010324 | ISBN 9781508185086 (library bound) | ISBN 9781508185079 (pbk.)
Subjects: LCSH: Radiologists—Juvenile literature. | Medical radiology—Vocational guidance—Juvenile literature. | X-rays—Juvenile literature.
Classification: LCC QC475.25 .P67 2019 | DDC 616.07/572/023—dc23
LC record available at https://lccn.loc.gov/2018010324

Manufactured in the United States of America

CONTENTS

INTRODUCTION 4

Chapter 1
LOOKING INTO RADIOLOGY 7

Chapter 2
RADIOLOGY DEPARTMENT ROLES 21

Chapter 3
AN EDUCATION IN RADIOLOGY 32

Chapter 4
GETTING HIRED 46

Chapter 5
PLOTTING A PROMISING CAREER 60

GLOSSARY 68
FOR MORE INFORMATION 70
FOR FURTHER READING 74
BIBLIOGRAPHY 75
INDEX 77

INTRODUCTION

Each day in a hospital's radiology department can be completely different from the day before. The day might start with routine checks of equipment to make sure everything is clean and in working order. After the patients start arriving, the work can be nonstop. It can be stressful and tiring, but also endlessly rewarding for the radiology technicians who work there.

Radiology technicians perform one of the most vital jobs in any hospital. They are thoroughly trained to use complex equipment to take images of the interior of people's bodies. These might be X-rays of fractured bones or CT scans for problems with the cardiovascular system. Their work is to create the images that can best help the doctors make a solid diagnosis and start treating the patient. This task involves positioning the patient and the machine to create the clearest image possible.

The work, however, is more than simply putting the patient in a machine and pressing buttons until an image is created. The radiology technician's job includes figuring out the best way to position the patient to create a clear image. He or she will describe the procedure to the patient and answer questions that come up. The radiology technician might have to calm the patient down so that the procedure can go ahead. Radiology technicians spend a full day repeating the process, though with

INTRODUCTION | 5

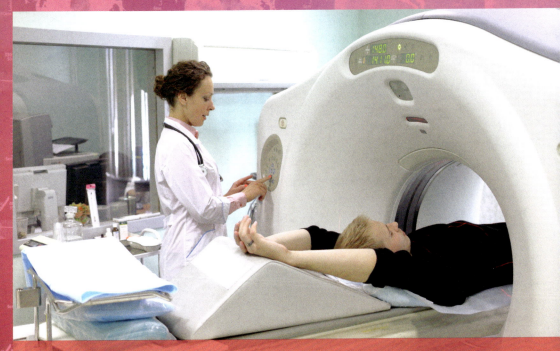

Radiology technicians care for patients of all ages as they go through imaging procedures. Here, a technician takes a boy through a magnetic resonance imaging (MRI) machine.

different patients. They'll see all kinds of people and encounter a wide variety of injuries and ailments.

Radiology technicians' training and their desire to help other people get better motivates them to perform well in their jobs. This training, which allows them to operate devices such as X-ray machines, can often be completed in fewer than two years at a community college or a hospital. Demand for radiology technicians is high, and the field is predicted to grow in the future. High school students who are interested in science and technology, and who have a strong desire to help people feel better, can expect to do well in the field.

After graduating and passing the necessary certification exams, a radiology technician is ready to begin a career in the field. Whether he or she focuses on one type of imaging device or earns the certifications needed to operate several types, there are numerous opportunities to produce high-quality images that can put patients on the road to recovery.

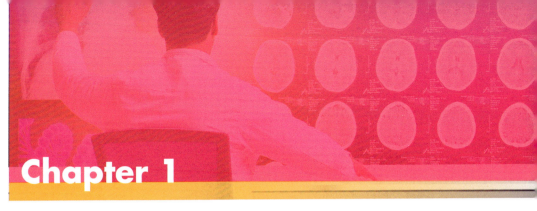

Chapter 1

LOOKING INTO RADIOLOGY

Radiology technicians are highly trained to use X-rays and sophisticated imaging equipment. Their work is vital to helping physicians and specialists find the cause of a patient's symptoms. In their work, they collect diagnostic information through visual images produced by complex machines. The images they collect may show bones, internal organs, soft tissues, or the cardiovascular system. From these images, physicians can find or rule out causes and get the patient on the right path to treatment.

Radiology is a complex field. Radiology technicians, sometimes called radiographers, must understand how the machines they use work, know how to capture the best images possible, and be able to put the patients they see at ease. Despite the importance of what they do and the high level of technical knowledge required, radiology technicians can be licensed after just two years of training.

Ready for Anything

Most radiological departments are located in hospitals, though there are some in private clinics or in imaging centers. Hospital radiological departments take care of all the imaging work for all of the departments. They handle patients coming in from the emergency room, oncology, maternity, gynecology, neurology, orthopedics, and other areas of practice. Because they see patients from all departments, radiological department staffers work with people of all ages.

The radiological department's function is to create images that are clear and can tell doctors everything they

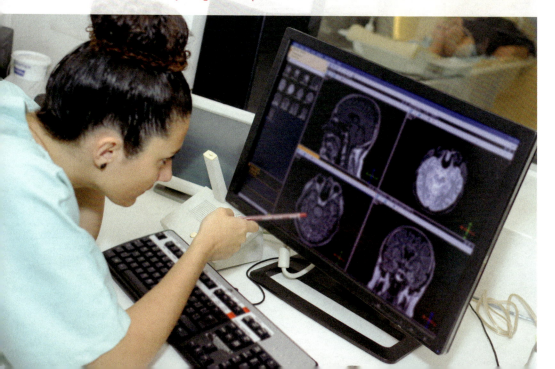

Obtaining clear images is vital to helping doctors decide on treatments. They should show the part of the body being treated from as many angles as possible.

need to know about the part of the body in question. Good, clear images will help doctors pinpoint fractures, tumors, blockages, and other causes of their patients' symptoms. An image might confirm the doctor's initial ideas about what's causing the symptoms, or it could reveal something totally unexpected. A series of images taken while a patient is being treated can show how he or she has responded to treatment.

Radiology technicians are the people who operate the machines, position the patients to provide the clearest possible images, and make high-quality prints of the images for the doctors to examine. They must be prepared to perform professionally and methodically in all cases. This means following an established series of steps to create the images and maintaining a good rapport with doctors and patients. They must be able to stay calm when they are under pressure to create images or when a patient is uncooperative. Regardless of what is happening around them, they have to create the best images possible.

Hours and Challenges

A hospital's radiology department operates around the clock. There are busy times during standard work hours, when the greatest number of doctors are in the hospital. However, there may be a need at any time for a patient to have an X-ray or other image taken. This demand is especially true of hospitals with emergency rooms, where patients may be coming in at all hours.

Radiology technicians may have to work irregular hours to meet the hospital's needs. Some technicians work evenings, while others work overnight. They may be on a permanent schedule that has them working the same hours from week to week, or they may have to switch from time to time. Techs must be flexible in making plans, finding a good sleep pattern, and planning meals and family time.

Radiology technicians should work to have a good rapport with the patients who come into their department. Many of these people are scared and nervous. Some may be in a great deal of physical pain. It's up to the radiology technician to put them at ease so that they feel comfortable during the imaging procedure. The radiology technician explains every part of the procedure,

Patients are often nervous or frightened before an imaging procedure. Radiology technicians can ease their fears by listening carefully, answering questions, and offering support.

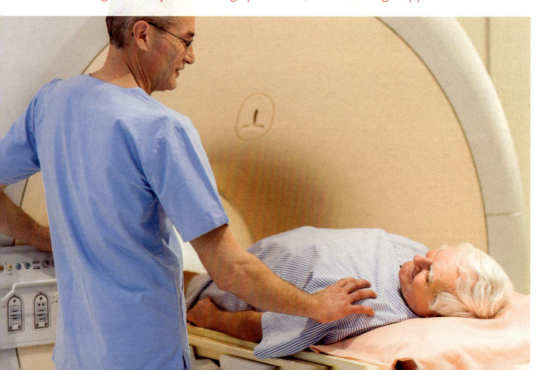

including how the patient will be asked to move if images from multiple angles are needed. He or she may answer questions about the type of equipment used, how long the process will take, and what happens after the imaging procedure.

Radiology technicians can't diagnose people or tell them about possible treatments. Although they are highly trained, they are not certified to offer medical opinions or give advice regarding the patient's treatment and probable outcome. They can advise patients to relax, reassure them that the imaging procedure they are about to undergo is safe, and let them know that the hospital's staff is committed to helping them get better.

Keeping that calm and reassuring manner can be difficult, especially after a long day and a heavy caseload. Some radiology technicians may find it hard to stay professional when spending their days seeing people suffering from serious injuries and illnesses. They must carefully balance their focus on their work with the need to act compassionately toward the patients they see.

Though the imaging machines they use are safe for patients, many of them do emit small doses of radiation. That radiation is in small enough doses that someone exposed to it for the length of time it takes to have an X-ray taken won't be harmed by it. Exposure over time, however, can damage a person's health. State health departments may have guidelines regarding how much radiation an employee can be exposed to over the course of a year.

Radiology technicians take measures to protect themselves. They may be required by law to wear lead aprons that are designed to block radiation. These aprons cover the entire torso and extend well past the waist. They may also have to wear dosimeters, which are devices that are designed to measure exposure to ionizing radiation, which is the kind of radiation used in imaging equipment. The small devices can track changes in exposure and cumulative exposure over time so that the radiology technician knows when he or she is approaching unsafe levels of exposure.

Knowing the Equipment

Radiology technicians work with highly specialized machines. Much of the equipment they work with is very advanced, large, and expensive. It's not unusual for a machine to cost hundreds of thousands of dollars. Some radiology technicians specialize in the use of one type of machine, though they may know how to use the other machines present in the department.

X-ray machines are the most widely used type of imaging equipment found in hospital radiology departments. They are also frequently found in clinics, private medical offices, and dentist's offices. X-ray technology has been around since 1895, when a German scientist named Wilhelm Roentgen discovered that electron beams could pass through cardboard to cast a light on the other side and could be used to capture an image of the bones of his hand. The process of using X-ray machines has changed very little since those days, though the machines themselves have evolved to become safer and more effective.

X-ray machines consist of a cathode and an anode that form an electron pair within a glass vacuum tube. An

LOOKING INTO RADIOLOGY | 13

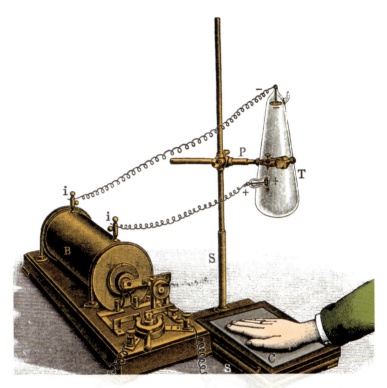

In this diagram of Roentgen's X-ray machine, a generator supplies electrical current that passes through a tube filled with a gas, creating electromagnetic rays that can produce images.

electrical current passes through the filament of the cathode to heat it up. This process causes electrons to be discharged from the filament. They are drawn by the positive anode, which is a disk made from the metal tungsten. The electrons collide with tungsten atoms, causing the release of a burst of energy called an X-ray photon. This energy is what passes through the patient's body to show an image of what's inside. Sometimes a chemical called a contrasting agent is put into the person's body so that problems are easier to spot.

The science behind creating X-rays has not changed much in the decades since Roentgen's discovery. The equipment used, however, has evolved greatly. For decades, the images created by X-ray machines were captured on film that had to be developed through a chemical process. Today, digital radiography eliminates the need for chemical development procedures, though many hospitals still use film for producing images. X-ray machines were once controlled manually but are now operated through computers. Technicians must be able to keep up with changes in the controls and operating systems. There are several kinds of X-ray machines that are used for specific purposes. They are specially designed to give physicians clear images of certain parts of the body or biological systems. Each requires specific knowledge and training.

Mammography machines use a very low-dose X-ray system to create highly detailed images of breast tissue called mammograms that are used to detect breast cancer in women. The technician positions the patient to produce the clearest image possible, then goes behind a wall to take the X-ray. Images are taken from several angles to pick up even the smallest tumor or abnormality.

Computerized tomography (CT) machines are imaging devices that produce a narrow band of X-rays that are rotated around a patient while he or she lies on a bed that moves slowly through a round opening in the machine. The rotating X-rays send signals to a computer, which processes this data to produce a series of digital images representing narrow slices of the patient's body. These tomographic images are more detailed than regular X-rays. They can be viewed individually or stacked

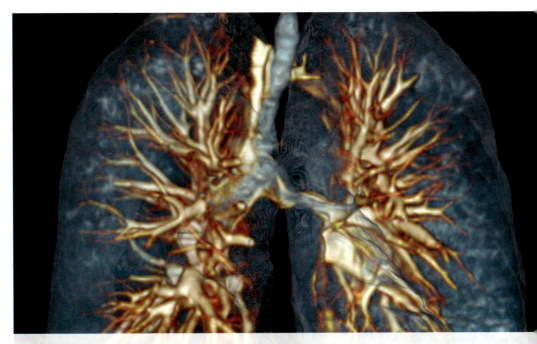

This color image from a computed tomography (CT) scan shows damage to lungs caused by emphysema (a disorder of the air sacs). The images can help doctors determine a course of treatment.

together to create a detailed three-dimensional (3D) representation of the patient. The 3D images show physical structures, such as the skeleton and organs, and can be rotated. This method gives doctors an easy way to identify possible tumors and other anomalies. Doctors may ask for a CT scan to identify tumors in the abdomen, hemorrhages in the head, heart blockages, fluid in the lungs, or other potentially life-threatening problems.

Unlike X-ray, mammography, and CT instruments, magnetic resonance imaging (MRI) instruments use

SONOGRAPHY AND ULTRASOUND

Radiology isn't the only field that involves medical imaging. Diagnostic medical sonographers, who work in the field of sonography, use ultrasound technology to visualize the internal structures of the body. Ultrasound machines work by directing high-frequency sound waves into the area of the body being scanned. An ultrasound machine does not utilize ionizing radiation, and for this reason, it is the standard image method used to image a fetus during pregnancy. There are many other specializations within sonography. Ultrasound procedures are well suited to imaging soft tissues of the body. Common specializations include imaging the abdomen, breast, musculoskeletal system, blood vessels, and heart. Pediatric sonographers specialize in imaging children and infants. Unlike radiological imaging procedures, sonography yields real-time images that can be viewed on a monitor as the sonographer is performing the procedure.

An associate's degree can prepare a sonographer for a career in the field, and the job outlook for sonographers is highly favorable. Technological advances have made sonography a safe, fast, and low-cost alternative to radiological scans in some circumstances. According to the Bureau of Labor Statistics (BLS) report in January 2018, employment of diagnostic medical sonographers is projected to grow 23 percent from 2016 to 2026, much faster than the average for all occupations. The BLS report also indicated that the median annual wage for diagnostic medical sonographers was $69,650 in 2016.

nonionizing magnetic radiation to create images. The use of this kind of device does not pose the same risk of cumulative radiation exposure as the other types of instruments.

As with CT instruments, a patient receiving an MRI scan lies flat on a bed that moves into the machine. Once inside the machine, powerful magnets generate enough energy to force the protons to line up with the magnetic field they create. A radiofrequency current is then sent through the patient that stimulates those protons and causes them to move around. When the current is turned off, the protons realign with the magnetic field. The speed at which they do this and the amount of energy they release can tell doctors about the types of tissues present. The machines can produce highly detailed images of soft tissues that are more difficult to capture with conventional X-rays.

Doctors use MRI instruments to check for problems in the brain, spinal cord, and nerves, where the ionized radiation released by CT scans might cause the most harm. They are also frequently used to spot problems with ligaments, muscles, and tendons. However, MRI scans are more expensive than CT scans or conventional X-rays.

A Fast-Paced Day

Whether they're working in a hospital radiology department, a clinic, or a private radiology practice, radiology technicians can expect to see patients with a wide range of medical problems. They may have to take X-rays or other diagnostic images of bone breaks, torn ligaments, or possible tumors. They may play a vital role in finding the cause of a patient's cough or the source of a persistent aching knee.

During the course of their workday, radiologists must perform many individual tasks. They check the equipment they'll be using to make sure it's working correctly. If necessary, they'll give the patient a fresh medical gown to wear during the imaging session. They'll talk with patients to make sure they are at ease with the procedure and to answer whatever questions they might have about it. They'll put the patient in the right position to take the best images possible. If the patient is disabled in some way, they may have to gently help get him or her in place.

Once the patient is in place, the radiology technician must make sure the patient isn't exposed to any unnecessary radiation. This step requires draping a lead-lined gown over the patient that covers vital organs and reproductive organs. The radiology technician then

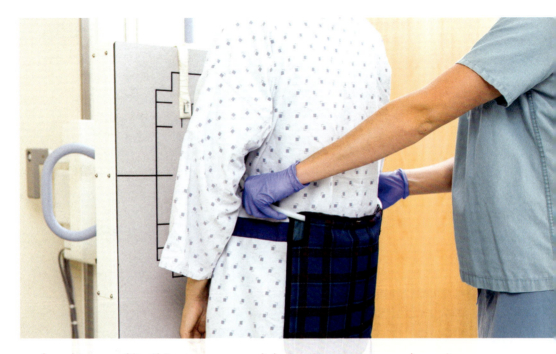

Lead aprons like this one are used during imaging procedures to protect patients from radiation that could potentially cause health problems later in life.

operates the machine—generally through a computer—to create an image. After the image is created—typically as a digital file but in some cases as film—the radiology technician examines it to make sure that it is clear and that it shows the doctor everything he or she needs to see to make a diagnosis.

A doctor may ask for more images to be taken from different angles, requiring the patient and sometimes the equipment to be repositioned. The radiology technician uses computer printing or chemical development processing techniques to make physical copies that can be studied. Prints may be blown up to focus on a small part of the area that is of concern. The radiology technician labels the prints and cross-references them with the patient's medical file so that they can be found easily if they are needed in the future. After that, it's time to clean up after the procedure. The table that the patient used and any equipment the tech handled is wiped down. If the patient wore a gown, it must be thrown away if it is made of paper or placed in a container to be sent to the laundry if it is fabric.

The time it takes to see a patient can depend on many factors, including the extent of the injury or medical condition, whether the physicians need multiple images taken, and whether the patient needs special assistance during the procedure. Some procedures may be scheduled by doctors in advance. Others may be slotted in around those previously scheduled sessions. As soon as one patient is done, another may be waiting.

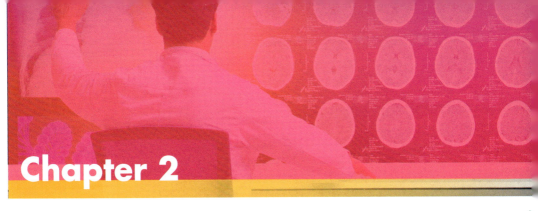

Chapter 2
RADIOLOGY DEPARTMENT ROLES

Health care workers who make radiology their specialty can fill a variety of important roles in a radiology department. The importance of X-rays, CT scans, and other images in making an accurate diagnosis means that the demand for skilled radiology specialists is unlikely to slow. Often, jobs within the field of radiology involve specialized knowledge of equipment and imaging techniques. A radiology technician may be trained and licensed to use a wide variety of imaging equipment but concentrate on one type of instrument, such as CT machines.

Radiology departments are typically overseen by a radiologist who is a board-certified physician. Although the radiologist is required to have a four-year degree and years of postgraduate medical training, four years of college is often not required for beginning a career in radiology. Most people who work in a radiology department need to earn only a two-year degree or complete a training program provided by an accredited institution.

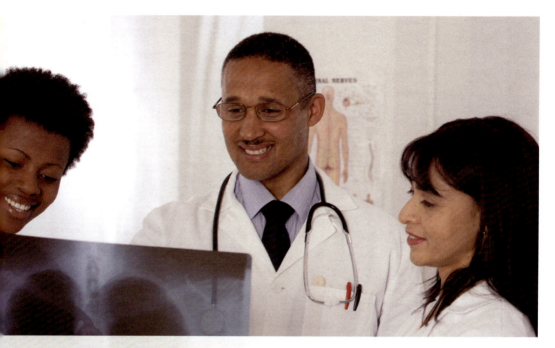

Radiology technicians and the radiologist who heads their department check X-rays for clarity. The radiologist can decide whether new images must be created.

Radiology Technicians

Radiology technicians are the backbone of any radiology department. They're the workers who are responsible for setting up, using, and maintaining the department's imaging equipment. They have to set the instruments' controls, make prints of the images, check the images for clarity, and deliver them to the physician. Radiology technicians not only get to use technologically advanced equipment but they also interact extensively with patients, nurses, and physicians.

The demand for radiology technicians is strong. According to the BLS report in January 2018, the median annual wage for a radiology technician was $58,960 in 2016. The outlook for the field is very positive. More radiology technicians are expected to be needed as the population ages and there are more instances of medical conditions that require imaging procedures. Employment for radiological technicians is expected to increase by 13 percent from 2016 to 2026, a faster rate than the average for all occupations.

Two-year degree or certificate programs are the typical education path for radiology technicians. Though professional certificates can be used to obtain a position as a radiological technician, that path is usually available only to those who have already earned a two-year associate's degree. These programs are available at most community colleges.

Students who want to become radiology technicians should have a strong interest in science, especially biology. Taking mathematics classes, physics courses, and anatomy classes are also recommended for high school students who think they want to work in radiology.

A real interest in the science and technology that are key to the profession can be invaluable. Radiology technicians must be ready to keep up with the latest developments in the field, especially new innovations in the technology regularly used in radiology departments and changes to professional guidelines. Radiology technicians should have an interest in helping improve people's lives. Classes in psychology can help future radiology technicians learn techniques for calming nervous patients and answering their questions in a reassuring way.

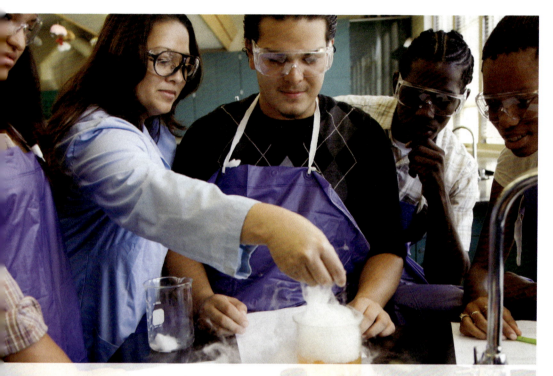

Doing well in high school science classes and enjoying lab work can be a sign that a student would like to work as a radiology technician.

Radiology technicians may specialize in using particular types of imaging devices. They likely must undergo additional training and be licensed to operate these machines. MRI technicians use the department or clinic's magnetic resonance imaging machines to capture three-dimensional, detailed images of the body's organs and tissues. For someone who already has experience in radiology or a two-year degree in the field, a certification program might take one or two years to complete at an institution accredited by the Joint Review

RADIOLOGY DEPARTMENT ROLES | 25

Becoming a mammographer requires additional training and education beyond what other radiology technicians receive. This specialization makes their skills highly desirable by hospitals and clinics.

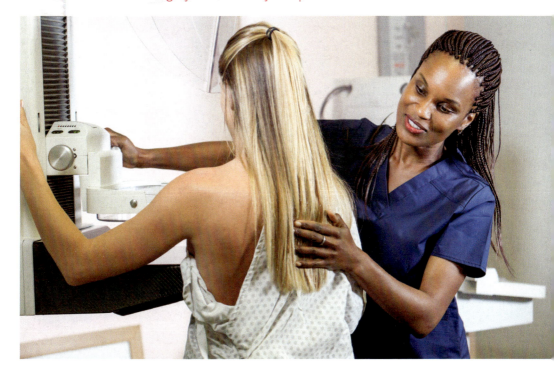

Committee on Education in Radiologic Technology. He or she would spend time in the classroom learning about the machines and reviewing anatomy and patient-interaction procedures. Prospective MRI technicians gain firsthand experience using MRI machines under the supervision of an instructor. They will also observe experienced MRI technicians at work. At the end of the program, they must take a certification exam given by the American Registry of Magnetic Resonance Imaging Technologists.

FINDING A CAREER IN RADIOLOGY

For Dennis Johnson, a certified radiologic technologist and computerized tomography supervisor at the National Institutes of Health in Bethesda, Maryland, it took a stint in the US Army to put him on his career path. In a profile on the job search website Monster.com, Johnson describes how he studied economics for two years at the New York City College of Technology before entering the military.

"During my time in the Army, I was trained as a radiologist," Johnson said in the profile. "The Army offered a licensing exam that I had to pass in order to practice my career. Once I passed it, I also took and passed the civilian exam, which allowed me to work in the civilian community." He later finished his economics degree and earned a master's degree in business administration but has continued to work in radiology.

"My typical workday is from 8 a.m. to 5:30 p.m. In our department, we see approximately 60 to 80 patients a day," Johnson said.

His duties include managing a staff of seven technicians and a patient coordinator, planning a budget, reviewing the workload and what each patient needs, consulting with staff radiologists, and maintaining and analyzing a patient database.

"We have three CT scanners that are busy all day long. Physicians schedule patients through the hospital information system. Then I receive the daily schedule and proceed with my responsibilities," Johnson said.

Johnson's favorite part of the job is interacting with patients. "Most of the patients that come through my department return for many years. I get to know them and their families. The best part of my job is to see a young patient grow up, and best of all, recover his or her health," he said in the profile.

To become a mammographer, a person must first earn a degree and certification in radiology. Next, he or she must complete forty hours of additional training focusing closely on mammography, as required by the US Food and Drug Administration. This training takes place under the direct supervision of a qualified instructor. The trainee learns about breast anatomy, how to position patients and compress tissue, how to properly use the equipment, and how to follow safety guidelines.

Candidates who make it through this part of the training must also perform at least twenty-five examinations under the supervision of a qualified instructor. They must also pass the mammography examination given by the American Registry of Radiologic Technologists (ARRT). The BLS classifies mammography technologists with radiology technicians. The statistical and salary data is the same for both on the BLS website.

Radiology technicians who specialize in CT/CAT scan procedures follow the same course of study as their peers. However, they are required to have verifiable experience using the machines in a clinical setting to perform specific procedures to receive professional certification. Additionally, for their first two years in the field they have to keep a record of the procedures they perform. The same BLS statistical data listed earlier also applies to these technicians.

Other Radiology Specialties

There are other career paths related to radiology that are open to students who want to be a part of the field. These jobs may require additional education or training. The people who perform them are invaluable members of the radiology department whose work helps everything run smoothly. Understanding their jobs can help radiology technicians understand their own roles in the department. These positions also give ambitious radiology technicians a goal to work toward if they're looking for ways to advance in the field.

Radiology assistants are radiology technicians who have undergone more education and certification. They work directly under the radiologists and can perform many of the same tasks, though only licensed radiologists

RADIOLOGY DEPARTMENT ROLES | 29

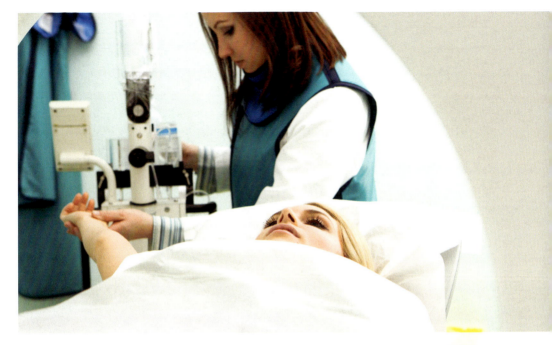

Radiology teams work hard to make sure their patients are ready for their procedures. Here, a contrast technician assists in preparing a woman for a CT scan.

are qualified to make a diagnosis. Radiology assistants have been trained to conduct tests, manage patients, and make preliminary judgments of test results. They handle many of the department's patient-care duties. These include patient assessments to determine whether the patient has been adequately prepared for the procedure. They'll get the patient's consent to undergo the procedure and answer questions.

The radiology assistant's main task is to see to it that the patient gets the highest quality of care possible. He or she may perform radiology procedures and exams under the radiologist's supervision. How much supervision is given may vary depending on the institution. He or she may serve as an important bridge between the radiologist and radiology technicians. Many of a radiology assistant's tasks help free up the radiologist to see to other parts of the job, such as analyzing images.

Radiology assistants must have earned at least a bachelor's degree from a four-year college or university, as well as received certification from the American Registry of Radiologic Technologists. They must pass an examination to prove that they are qualified to be employed as radiologic assistants and keep up with

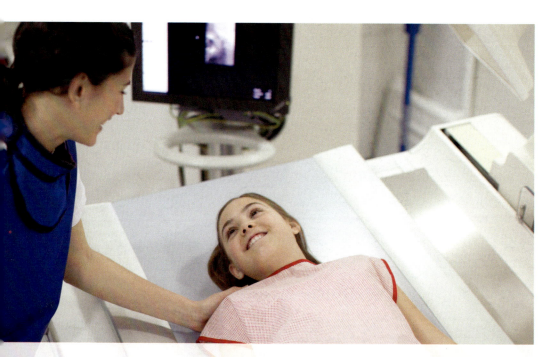

Making sure patients of all ages are comfortable and relaxed before an imaging procedure begins is a key part of a radiology nurse's job.

continuing education requirements in order to hold onto their ARRT registration.

Radiology nurses are registered nurses who have gone through additional training to work with patients in radiology departments. Their primary job is to supervise the patients' recovery from imaging procedures and make sure they are comfortable. Preparing to become a radiology nurse takes a great deal of time. Students must complete at least a two-year nursing degree, though many radiology nurses have bachelor's degrees or even master's degrees.

Once they have a nursing degree, prospective radiology nurses must sign up for and pass an exam called the NCLEX-RN, which tests practical knowledge and a nurse's ability to respond to a wide variety of situations. Exam questions might cover topics such as home safety, crisis intervention, continuity of care, cultural awareness, and resource management. Finally, nurses must work as registered nurses within a radiology department for at least two thousand hours and receive an additional thirty hours of education in radiology to be able to take the certification exam.

Chapter 3

AN EDUCATION IN RADIOLOGY

Most jobs within the radiology department require only a two-year degree or less, with the exception of the more specialized positions of radiology nurse, radiologist, and radiological assistant. There are several types of institutions that provide training in radiology. Community colleges, vocational schools, private institutions, or hospitals themselves offer programs that can give students interested in radiology the training they need to succeed in the field.

Laying a Framework

Interested students can start laying the foundation for a career in radiology in middle school or high school. The basic building blocks begin with an interest in science and math, as well as a strong desire to help people.

Any training program in radiology requires students to hold a high school diploma or its equivalent. Interested students should begin by studying science subjects such as biology, chemistry, and physics. Doing well in these classes can help prepare you for training after graduation and give you an idea of whether you truly are interested in pursuing a career that depends so much on scientific knowledge.

Other classes that can be helpful include algebra and trigonometry. The math classes are important for calculating the proper position for imaging equipment during a procedure. Psychology classes can be useful for finding effective ways of communicating with nervous or frightened people. Understanding why patients might be worried or uncomfortable can help radiology technicians relax them.

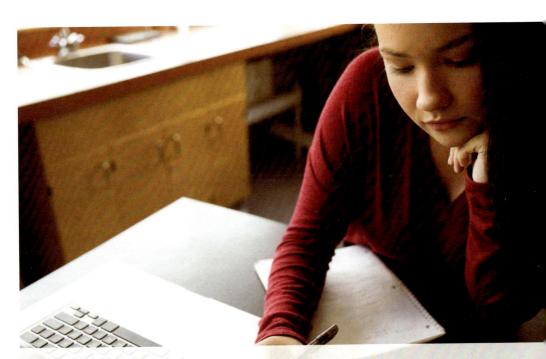

Radiology technicians must be able to do mathematical calculations quickly and accurately to create the best images possible. Understanding algebra is necessary to doing the job well.

Some health care systems and hospitals offer summer internships that give high school students the opportunity to observe medical professionals in action and gain some hands-on experience. Often, these internships are open to students entering their junior or senior years, as well as to graduating seniors. Participants may be able to earn college credit through these internships, depending on the program. The National Institutes of Health, the Rochester Institute of Technology, and Southern Illinois Healthcare are among the institutions, schools, and organizations that welcome high school students as interns.

Helpful Traits

People who are looking into a career in radiology should have a strong desire to help people improve their lives and their health. They will likely be working with people from all age groups and backgrounds, so they must be comfortable relating to people with whom they might not have much in common on the surface. Solid communication skills and a sense of compassion can equip radiology technicians for full days of working with patients. They should be able to communicate effectively with the people they see, while taking into account their feelings and worries.

Radiology technicians also must be attentive to detail and careful in their work habits. They should be willing to take the time to make sure they have the right angles for lining up their equipment and that the patient is comfortable while waiting for the procedure to be completed. If the radiologist or other doctors need to have more images made, the technician should be prepared to do so to the specifications given. A good image can be the key to diagnosing a serious illness or helping doctors find the right treatment for an injury. A bad image could hide helpful information and delay the patient's treatment or lead to an incorrect diagnosis and treatment.

Careful work habits can help radiological technicians follow the correct procedures every time. Someone who is accustomed to following a specific series of steps can do well in the field. Radiology technicians should also be attentive to their equipment and their department's environment. Keeping things clean and sterile is a must. Cleaning and caring for the equipment should come as second nature. Radiological technicians must notice when

Caring for delicate imaging equipment is a major part of a radiology technician's job. Students learn how to keep it working properly and how to spot potential problems.

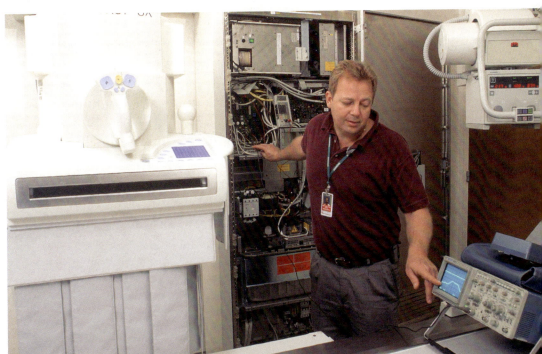

their imaging equipment is malfunctioning and be able to pinpoint the problem. Many technicians can perform some repairs themselves, as well as general maintenance tasks. The equipment they use is expensive, sensitive, and vital to treating patients. Any misuse or time that it is inoperable can have life-threatening consequences to patients.

Patient safety is another area where radiology technicians need to pay attention. The ionizing radiation released by imaging machines can cause significant health problems if the dosage is too high. Radiology technicians should always be aware of the amount of radiation to which their patients are being exposed, as well as how much they themselves are absorbing.

The care needed in tending to patients is also needed for taking care of the valuable equipment used in imaging. Radiology technicians are responsible for keeping equipment clean and sterile, including the beds patients are asked to lay on when going through a CT or MRI machine. Surfaces must be thoroughly disinfected and wiped down before another patient can come through for a procedure. Radiology technicians themselves will wear a fresh pair of gloves for each procedure.

Training Options

A person interested in studying for a career in radiology may be faced with numerous options from which to choose. The ARRT lists more than 1,400 accredited institutions in the United States that offer programs in radiography. More than half of those programs are offered by hospitals. These programs are two-year certificate or diploma programs that include classroom time and hands-on learning in a clinic environment, where students interact directly with patients and perform procedures under supervision.

In an article titled "Advice for Getting Hired as a Radiologic Technologist" by the website Radiology Schools 411, Michigan Society of Radiologic Technologists president Cindy Reszke recommended that students can benefit from learning to take constructive criticism well and learning from every situation during those clinic sessions.

"I feel that the best advice to getting hired as a radiologic technologist is to treat your clinical education as a job interview. The programs are long and very demanding, but it is important to consistently put your best effort forward," Reszke said.

Community colleges offer about 40 percent of the accredited programs available. These are two-year associate's degree programs. As with the hospital programs, community college students are exposed to a mix of classroom time and hands-on learning experiences designed to help them become used to real-life situations they might face in a radiology department.

There are some vocational schools that offer one-year certification programs for professionals such as registered nurses and medical technologists who may work with the department, though they are not directly involved in the imaging process at any point. Universities offer four-year bachelor's or two-year master's degrees for those interested in supervisory roles or teaching positions.

Students attend classes full-time in all these programs. They must become deeply familiar with the machines they'll be using, medical terminology, and the human body to succeed in the field. Although they don't treat or consult with patients, their education includes anatomy. They'll learn about bone structure and locations of vital organs and become familiar with the cardiovascular and nervous systems. This instruction enables them to fully understand what the physicians want when they get their patients ready for an imaging procedure. With a thorough understanding of anatomy, students can have a better idea of how to position a patient to produce high-quality images.

Radiation physics courses help prospective radiology technicians understand how energy is emitted or transmitted through space or a physical medium. They'll study the ionizing radiation that make X-rays an effective

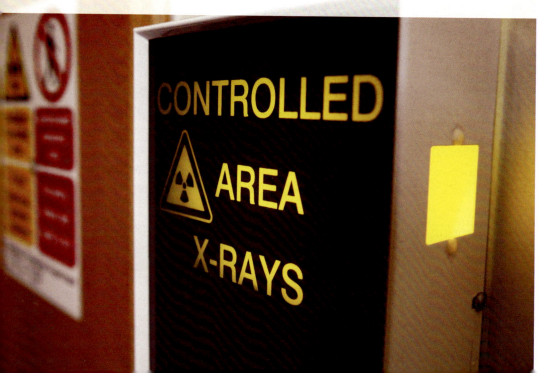

Radiation can cause serious health problems in radiology technicians and patients. To keep people safe, hospitals and clinics restrict access to areas where it is used.

imaging tool. They'll learn how to safely use imaging equipment and how to protect themselves from overexposure to potentially harmful radiation.

Medical ethics classes examine the ethical questions that arise from efforts to improve public health. Students learn about topics such as the rights of patients, genetic testing, and experimenting on people. Radiation technicians won't directly encounter many of those complex situations in their work, but they may have to handle cases in which a patient refuses a procedure, for example.

"Take advantage of every opportunity given during your time in school," Joel Hicks, clinical coordinator of the Radiologic Science Program and assistant professor at the School of Allied Health at Northwestern State University, told Radiology Schools 411. "This can be everything from CPR classes to fulfilling requirements to take a CT or MR registry. Employers want employees who can step in and work. Everything that you can provide that will keep you from losing time will be a benefit to your employer and ultimately, to you."

Students in radiology programs offered by hospitals are likely to have numerous opportunities for hands-on learning. However, those in community college or technical schools will need to look for internships that give them on-the-job training in a hospital or clinic setting. Interns will likely have firsthand opportunities to operate imaging equipment while following the protocols of the hospital where they're working. Though they may serve out their internship as an assistant to a specialist, such as an MRI technician, it's likely that they'll be asked to rotate through the department to gain experience with other equipment and procedures.

GAINING NEW SKILLS

Although many radiology technicians specialize in using specific types of imaging equipment, some professionals in the field recommend that students learn as much as possible about a wide range of imaging devices to increase their chances of getting hired.

Sandra Hayden, vice president of the American Society of Radiologic Technologists, advises that students who have trained on just one type of equipment seek out mentors who can help them learn more about different imaging devices. Hayden told Radiology Schools 411 the following:

> You can also go to the vendor's website, as they often have links to videos and educational tools. Look for opportunities to observe new equipment and become familiar with its benefits and drawbacks. Hiring someone with prior knowledge and experience makes it easier for an employer because they won't have to spend as much time and resources training you. Knowing their equipment and systems gives you an edge over the competition.

> **An employer's hiring manager often will seek to fill positions with those who already have hands-on experience with the equipment that is necessary for that particular job.**

To succeed as interns, radiology students must show that they can work well in a clinical setting and accomplish all of their assigned tasks. They'll have to demonstrate competency in using imaging machines under supervision and in working with patients. They'll also have to show that they have the medical and anatomical knowledge to follow a physician's directions, as well as the analytical skills to position the patient and equipment in the best way possible. A professional appearance; team-oriented attitude; good time management skills; and ability to work cooperatively with physicians, staff members, and patients can make an internship a rewarding experience.

Internships may take place in limited hours during the semester or with close to full-time hours during the summer, depending on the hospital. Some interns are paid an hourly wage or a weekly or monthly stipend. Others are unpaid. Still others provide college credit for your work. You may need to meet certain education requirements to work in some radiology internships. Look for internships that offer the pay options and hours that best fit your needs. Keep in mind that internships can sometimes lead to job offers. It's not unusual for an intern who performs well in that role to be offered a full-time position on condition of completing his or her degree and getting certified.

Earning Certification

Earning a two-year diploma or a professional certificate is not enough to find work in radiology after graduating. Even entry-level radiology technologist positions require that the applicant have professional certification. By earning certification, graduates of radiology programs prove that they have the knowledge needed to operate imaging equipment, take care of patients, and follow safety procedures.

Certification is provided by the ARRT. The organization offers credentials in imaging technology, as well as radiation therapy and other procedures. The ARRT's examination for radiologists is more than three hours long and features 220 questions covering a wide range of topics, including procedures for operating equipment, patient-care practices, creating images, and radiation physics. They'll be asked questions about things like patient management and proper procedures for creating images of extremities.

Multiple-choice questions that an ARRT's certification test taker might face include "What is a myocardial infarction?" or "Which of the following are subatomic particles?" The questions might ask about specific bones, chemicals used in some procedures, or how to handle patients with specific medical needs.

Passing the exam is necessary for anyone hoping to secure even an entry-level position as a radiation technologist. Although attending classes and earning a degree will give you the educational background needed to do well on the test, it is also important to study in the weeks leading up to the exam itself. Because so much material may be covered, reviewing even basic material might be necessary. Talking to people who have passed the exam can help you formulate strategies for succeeding. The ARRT outlines the four criteria that are covered on the exam: patient care, safety, image production, and procedures.

Some companies offer question banks designed to help test takers prepare for the exam. Signing up for a question bank will cost money, but it gives you access to a wide selection of practice questions that you can use to create your own mock exams for testing how your studies are progressing. Some question bank suppliers offer thorough explanations for the correct answers, giving you the chance to fully understand the topic. You'll be able to see how your scores improve and identify areas where you need improvement.

Developing a smart test-taking strategy for the exam can also help you succeed. The fact that the exam is timed and features hundreds of questions can be intimidating. Set limits for how long you'll allow yourself to think about each question to avoid getting stuck. If that time passes, eliminate the answers that you know are wrong and make the best guess you can on those that remain. That way, you can move ahead in the exam knowing that you increased your chances of answering correctly. This strategy can also help you remain focused during the test and answer questions you do know with confidence.

Preparing for a test should include spending some time answering mock test questions while working against a time limit. This technique can help students overcome nervousness on test day.

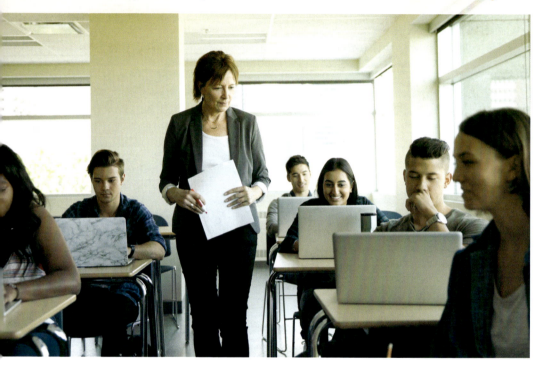

Preparing for getting to the exam itself can help eliminate a major source of stress and free you to concentrate on the test itself. Figure out what you're going to wear the night before and have your clothes ready. The ARRT requires that test takers show two forms of identification at the site, so have those prepared as well. Plan out exactly how you'll get to the testing site, including mapping out your route and figuring out what room you'll need to go to when you get there. If you're driving, be sure your car is ready to go. If you're taking public transportation or a taxi or ride-sharing service, make sure you have the appropriate fare ready. Plan to leave home early so that you'll still be on time in case you encounter any delays. Getting there half an hour early will give you time to present your identification, have your palm scanned, get a photo taken, and offer a digital signature, all of which are required by the ARRT. Also, be sure to get a good night's sleep and have something to eat before you leave for the test. Being tired or hungry may throw you off and keep you from getting the best score possible.

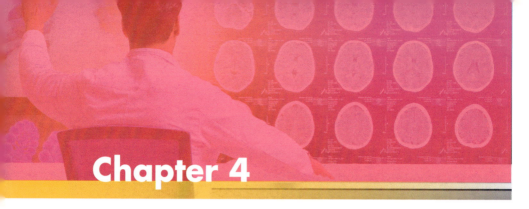

Chapter 4
GETTING HIRED

Radiology technicians are in demand in hospitals, clinics, imaging centers, and private practice offices. A well-trained and prepared graduate who has earned certification in radiology should be able to find a job through persistence and with the help of resources such as job fairs, networking opportunities, and online postings.

Selling Your Skills

Composing a résumé should be one of the first steps a recent graduate makes before starting a job hunt or even before graduating. A résumé is a short document that describes a person's educational background, employment history, and any special skills or professional certifications that he or she has accumulated. Students who have applied for internships have likely created résumés. Some summer jobs or college work-study positions may also require a résumé.

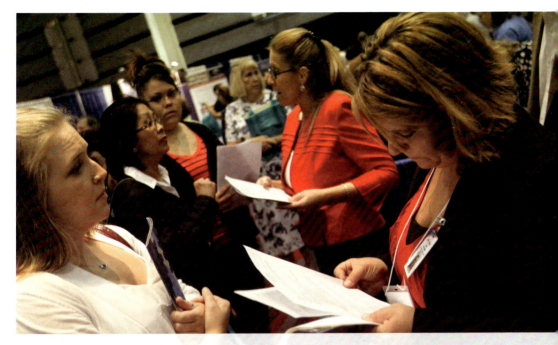

Job fairs give students a chance to show their résumé to recruiters, who can sometimes offer advice on how job seekers present their qualifications.

Recent high school or community college graduates likely will not have very lengthy résumés. Theirs will probably show which schools they attended and when they graduated or expect to graduate. It will highlight their major or concentration, such as radiology, and may list some of the courses they took to highlight particular specialties.

Details such as club memberships, extracurricular activities, internships, and volunteer work will be

48 | JUMP-STARTING A CAREER IN RADIOLOGY

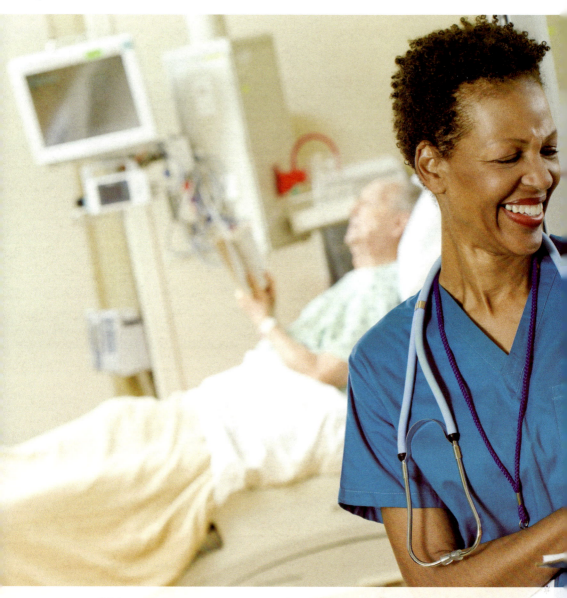

Volunteer programs at hospitals give students interested in working in medicine the chance to perform hands-on duties. A nurse explains a procedure to a teen volunteer.

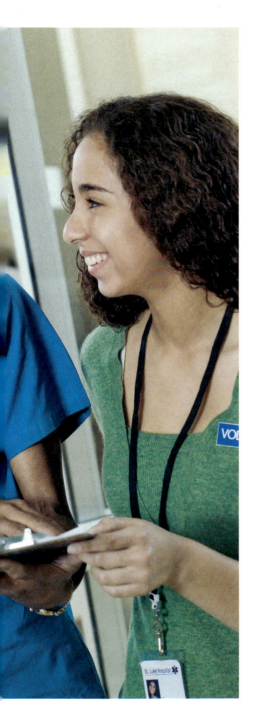

described to show that the applicant has a well-rounded and engaged personality. If the applicant was chosen to take part in an honors program or studied abroad, that information should also be included.

Résumés don't simply go to employers to be filed away. Recruiters study them closely to see if the applicant has experience that is relevant to the job or shows an ability to take on new challenges. They'll look for structural details in the résumé itself, including the way it is organized and formatted. They'll check to make sure all the information presented in the document is factually accurate. Recruiters even look for serious spelling and grammatical errors as a way to check whether the applicant is attentive to such details.

Even the way in which applicants describe their work and educational experience can affect the results of a job application. Recruiters tend to look for résumés that use an active voice to describe accomplishments and tasks, rather than those that simply list experiences. Résumés should also be as current as possible. If the applicant is working at a job or an internship at the time, it should also be included.

Composing good cover letters gives you a way to tell recruiters more about yourself than they may get from the résumé alone. Most cover letters are only a page long, but they provide applicants with a chance to offer specific examples of why they might be well suited for a job. It's important to avoid simply repeating the information that's on your résumé and instead describe ways you've used your knowledge or skills. A radiology technician might describe instances in which he or she helped with a difficult patient, for example. As with résumés, recruiters look at the way the cover letter is constructed, check that they are factually accurate, and make note of any major grammatical or spelling errors. They will also notice if the letter is obviously a generic template that's being sent out to multiple employers. It helps to specifically cite ways in which your experience relates directly to the position for which you're applying and to mention the prospective employer in the letter.

Using Resources

Schools often have career centers that can help students and recent graduates focus their job search. The people who work there are trained to help students find jobs or internships in their fields of study. They can help you narrow your search and suggest prospective employers. They may be in touch with other graduates who have found work in radiology and are able to set up interviews or calls with their employers. Career centers can also help students fine-tune their résumés. They'll review the documents and offer tips on how to make them stronger, as well as point out any obvious errors that could have a negative impact on the job search.

Many schools participate in job fairs, in which prospective employers set up booths or tables. Representatives of the hospital or clinic will be there to discuss job openings and answer questions about their workday, job benefits, and important factors that can help you decide whether a position there is right for you. Pick up any brochures or other information they may have so that you can compare their information with that from other potential employers. Be sure to have copies of your résumé with you to offer to representatives from employers that you feel would be a good fit. The recruiters who attend job fairs often have business cards on hand that you can take with you in case you want to get in touch with them about future job opportunities. You may be able to sign up for an email list that will include you in future outreach efforts when more jobs become available.

Some public library systems offer programs for job hunters. They may have career counselors come in to help people focus their job searches, offer tips for getting through a job interview, and review résumés and cover letters. A library may also offer books designed

JUMP-STARTING A CAREER IN RADIOLOGY

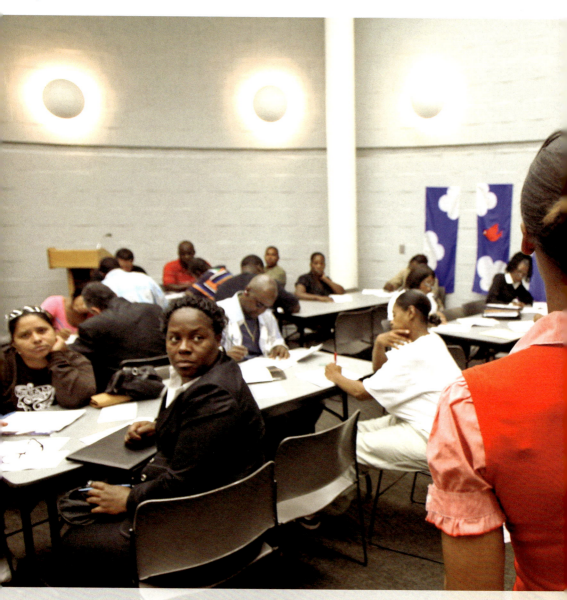

Hospitals with openings in high-demand areas such as radiology may hold job fairs in major cities to attract seasoned professionals looking for new employment opportunities.

GETTING HIRED | 53

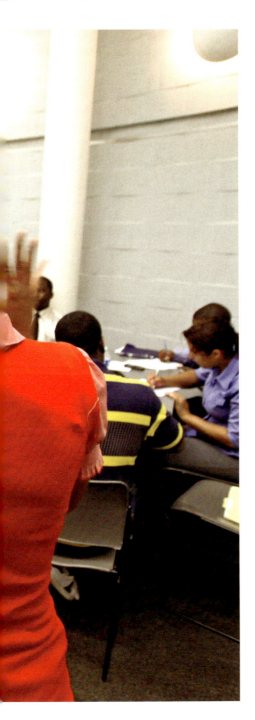

to help applicants study for exams or that list prospective employers, including hospitals and clinics.

There are many job search websites, including some that specialize in health care careers. Be sure to check both general job search websites as well as health care job sites for positions that could be right for you. Major job-hunting sites such as CareerBuilder, Indeed, and Monster list jobs in the health care industry that can be narrowed by state, city, or town. Hospitals may advertise for radiology technicians in newspapers and professional journals. Online message boards can be another good spot to look for job openings in the field. Seek out job listings from hospitals themselves. Many hospitals with radiology departments will list any openings they need to fill on their websites. The same is true of clinics.

Radiology-specific websites may also offer job listings. Professional organizations such as the American College of Radiology give members access to recent job postings from hospitals across the United States. Search for positions in your area or explore opportunities in other places if you're willing to move for your career.

Networking in Radiology

Maintaining a strong network with your classmates, teachers, and people you meet during your internship can be invaluable to finding a good job in radiology. Former classmates who are already working in the field can keep you informed of any new openings at their places of employment.

Developing a strong and supportive network of classmates, instructors, and mentors can begin even before graduation. You may form strong bonds with your classmates as you work toward your degree or certificate. Those connections can serve you well when you begin your job search. People you work with during an internship and faculty members at your school can also be helpful when you're looking for job opportunities. Don't be afraid to reach out to alumni who have graduated from your radiology program. They may have positions that they need to fill in their radiology departments and may be willing to hire talented graduates of their old schools. Professors may be in touch with many of these former students and might be able to help you make those valuable professional connections.

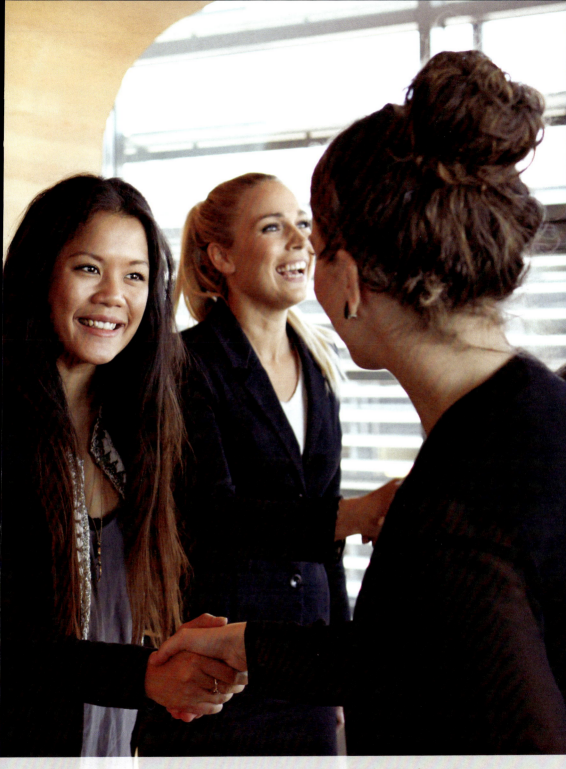

Networking gives job seekers the chance to talk about job openings, discuss the benefits of working for certain employers, and pass along helpful information.

CREATING A NETWORK

Developing a network of colleagues, teachers, and employers who can help you on your career path in radiology takes work. Joy A. Cook, president of the Indiana Society of Radiologic Technologists, advises that students begin networking as soon as possible, including going beyond their classrooms to join organizations associated with radiology. The people students meet during this networking process may be able to point them in the right direction for finding a job or even be in a position to hire them.

Cook told Radiology Schools 411:
When students take full advantage of becoming members of their local, state, or national professional organizations they have the opportunity to start meeting and networking with individuals already in the field of imaging sciences.

Cook also advised that the clinic portion of the radiology program is an important networking opportunity. Each clinic or staff rotation a student spends time in offers new chances to make a good impression and create strong professional connections.

Cook said:
While clinical work is part of the educational process, it also might be the start

of a yearlong interview as the facilities students practice in may be looking to hire upon graduation. During clinical education students want to show those they work around, with, and for their best personality and work traits; it might be the difference between a job interview or the job offer."

The Interview Process

Job interviews can be extremely stressful, but there are steps you can take to help reduce that stress. A good place to start is to consider the invitation to the interview as a small victory. Remember that out of all the candidates who applied for a particular job, you were one of the few chosen to go in for an interview.

Plan ahead as much as you can in the days before the interview. Learn all you can about the hospital or clinic where you would be working, including any areas of specialization, such as oncology care or pediatrics. Find out what you can about specific requirements and responsibilities that are part of the job.

Develop responses to questions that the interviewer might ask, such as why you feel you're the candidate who's best qualified for the job and what you might expect from the job. You'll also want to prepare some questions of your own about the job, the work environment, and the types of cases you're likely to see. You might ask about the types of imaging equipment the

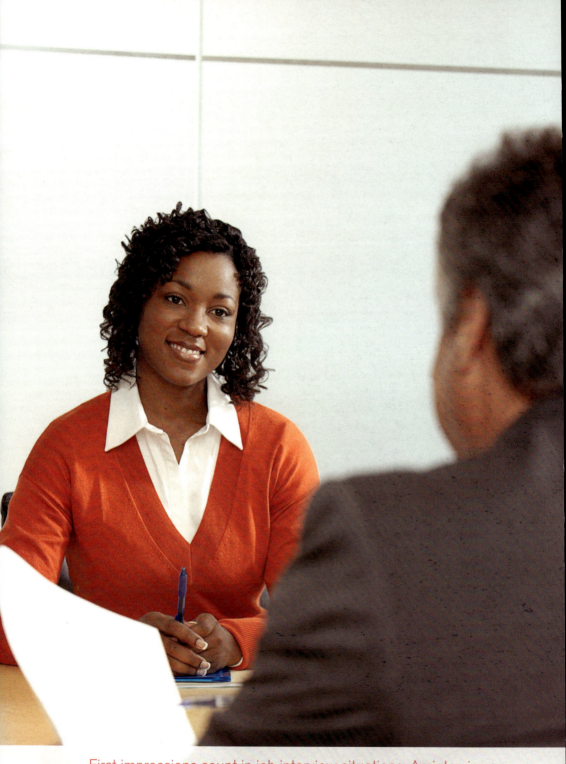
First impressions count in job interview situations. An interviewer may make judgments about a candidate's fitness for a position based on whether he or she looks and acts professionally.

department has as a way to show that you're genuinely interested in the job.

Presenting yourself in a positive light is vital to success in a job interview. Make sure that you'll be on time. Punctuality is invaluable in radiology, and you want to show that you can be where you're needed at the right time. Plan your route to the interview and give yourself enough time to allow for traffic or other problems. It never hurts to arrive a little early so that you have time to tidy up and gather your thoughts.

Choose a professional-looking outfit to wear and set it out the night before so that it will be ready. Dressing well shows that you take the interview process seriously and demonstrates respect for the interviewer. During the interview itself, try to be confident, polite, and friendly. Giving honest and articulate answers to the interviewer's questions will show that you understand the job you would be doing and that you take it seriously enough to give thoughtful responses. Projecting competence and a positive attitude demonstrates that you have the knowledge needed to do the work and the demeanor to handle stressful situations.

After the interview is over, send a message to the interviewer thanking him or her for the opportunity to discuss the job. Avoid asking whether you're likely to be hired until a few days have passed, and only if you have not been contacted by anyone about your status. If everything goes well, you might hear back and either be called in for a second interview or offered the job.

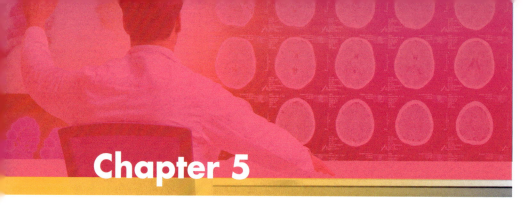

Chapter 5

PLOTTING A PROMISING CAREER

After you are hired for your first job in a radiology department, it may seem as though you've completed all the steps you need to take in planning your career. However, radiology is a growing field and there are many opportunities available to grow professionally and develop new skills. Radiology technicians who show they have a strong work ethic and an ability to learn new responsibilities can advance in their department or potentially look for better opportunities at other hospitals and clinics. With additional training and education, a radiology technician can become proficient in the use of more types of imaging machines. With every new skill added, the radiology technician becomes an even more valuable part of the department. With more education, a position as a radiology assistant or even as a radiologist may be an attainable goal.

PLOTTING A PROMISING CAREER | 61

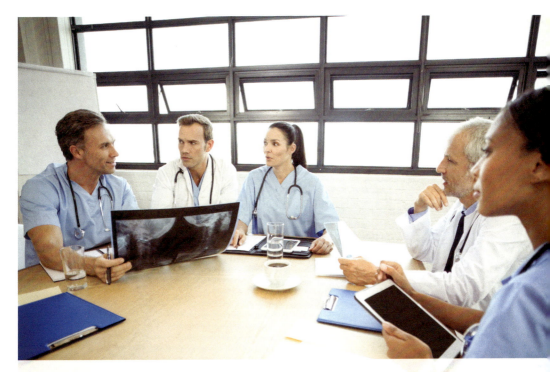

Radiology technicians may decide that they want a bigger role in medicine. Working in radiology can prepare them for beginning training in other career areas or leadership roles.

Becoming Invaluable

Your first job as a radiology technician will probably be an entry-level position. Even if you got good grades in your classes and completed a demanding internship, the radiologist and more experienced radiology technicians will probably keep a close eye on your work for the first several weeks or even months. Radiology is a field in which even small mistakes can have enormous

62 | JUMP-STARTING A CAREER IN RADIOLOGY

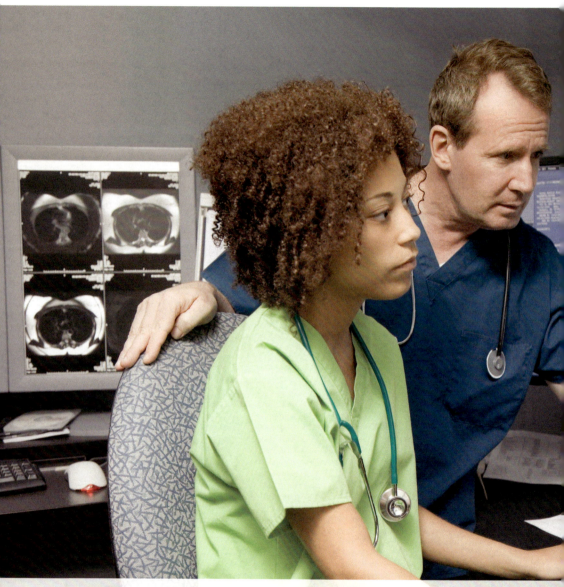

Training prepares radiology technicians for many situations they'll face on the job. They'll continue learning as they work with more experienced employees who can give expert guidance.

PLOTTING A PROMISING CAREER

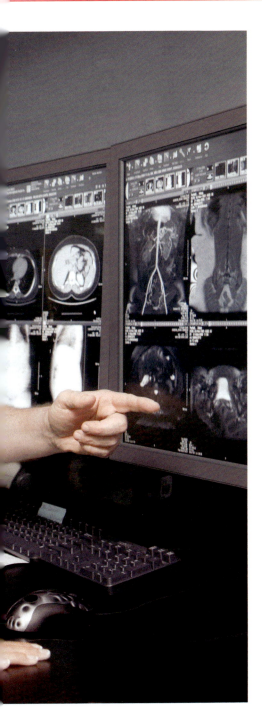

consequences for patients. They'll want to make sure that any errors you make are caught quickly or minimized to prevent the patient from being harmed.

Be sure to listen to constructive criticism from other members of the department. They almost certainly have more experience than you, and you can probably learn a great deal from them about imaging procedures and interacting with patients. Don't be afraid to ask questions if you don't understand why something is done in a certain way or if you're having trouble. Everyone in the department wants to help patients get better, and all want to make sure that you understand what you're doing so that you can help achieve that goal. Showing that you can be counted on to be on time and where you're needed can help demonstrate that you're motivated to do the best job possible and help the department.

REWARDS OF THE JOB

A visit to the radiology department is often an important step in a patient's journey back to good health. Without the detailed images radiology technicians provide, physicians might not be able to develop a proper course of treatment.

For Jeremy Enfinger, the radiology lead tech at Scripps Health, in San Diego, California, working with a wide range of different people is one of the best parts of the job, as he told the website Carestream. Other rewarding aspects of the field for Enfinger included the artistic element of creating images, the flexibility of the field, and the technology itself. Enfinger also said he appreciates the camaraderie of working in radiology.

Enfinger said in the interview:

After a few short years, I genuinely feel like I know someone in every hospital for at least a 100 mile radius. It's a very small world in radiography, and that world seems even smaller the more time you spend in the field.

You'll also want to prove that you can get along well with your supervisors, coworkers, and patients. If you like your job well enough to want to stay there for a few years, you'll have to be able to work well with everyone else. Even if you don't want to stay that long, you may want to use your coworkers or supervisors as references. You might be more likely to get hired for another position if they can honestly say that you interacted well with others and served as a valuable part of the team.

Advancing in the Field

Be sure to look for ways in which you can grow professionally. There may be opportunities to train on different types of equipment while you're working. Some hospitals will partially reimburse your tuition if you're taking classes that can add to your skills as a medical professional. You may even be able to take classes toward certification in specializations like MRI or mammography imaging at your hospital. Take advantage of those opportunities to expand your skills. The more certifications you have, the more in-demand your skills will be and you'll qualify for higher wages.

Identify areas that you're strong in and try to add certifications to your résumé. A CT/CAT scan certification can open up new possibilities for you in the event that you want to look for a position elsewhere. The same is true with mammography certification or working as a sonographer. You might also consider continuing your education. A position as a radiologist, a radiology assistant, or a radiology nurse might interest you and provide more chances for growth in the field.

66 | JUMP-STARTING A CAREER IN RADIOLOGY

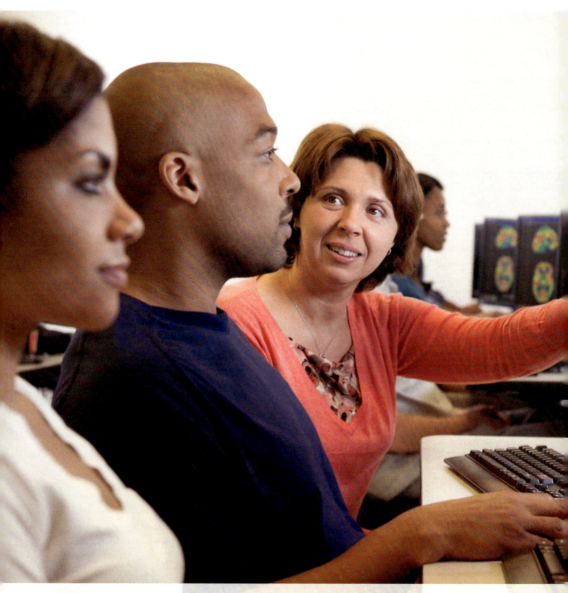

Experienced radiology technicians who have multiple certifications can bring many skills and a broad range of knowledge to a radiology team, making them highly desirable employees.

PLOTTING A PROMISING CAREER | **67**

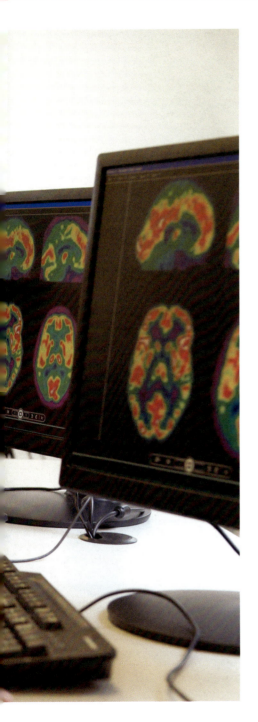

As you work in the field and build on your skills, continue to network. Keep in touch with former colleagues, supervisors, and employers. They may be able to help you with a reference or a letter of recommendation in the future. Staying close to fellow students and teachers can also prove valuable as you navigate your career in radiology.

GLOSSARY

accredited Describing an organization, course of study, or employee that has been officially approved.

associate's degree A degree awarded to a student who has completed a two-year program at a community college, college, or university.

bachelor's degree The undergraduate degree obtained after completing a four-year college program.

cardiovascular Related to or involving the heart and blood vessels.

certification The awarding of a certificate or license upon completion of a course of study or passing of an exam.

diagnose To identify the nature of a medical condition by examining the symptoms.

extremity A part of the body that is distant from the main part, such as a hand.

imaging The process of using a machine to create an image by passing an electronic beam over something.

internship A short-term training job, generally completed to gain practical experience.

license Official permission from the government or other authority, such as to practice a trade.

network To maintain communication with a group of people, especially to exchange information about professional opportunities.

oncology The branch of medical science that deals with preventing, diagnosing, and treating cancers and tumors.

procedure A series of steps carried out in a particular way in order to complete a task.

rapport A relationship of understanding, trust, and respect between two people.
recruiter A person who seeks out qualified workers to hire for a particular job.
reference Someone providing a statement of professional qualifications; also, the statement itself.
résumé A summary of one's professional qualifications and work experience.
stipend A certain amount of money paid for work done or to cover expenses.
technician Someone trained in practical application and knowledge, especially of a mechanical or scientific subject.
vendor An individual or company that sells goods and services.
X-ray A photograph produced by certain electromagnetic radiation waves.

FOR MORE INFORMATION

American College of Radiology
1891 Preston White Drive
Reston, VA 20191
(703) 648-8900
Website: https://www.acr.org
Facebook: @AmericanCollegeOfRadiology
Twitter: @RadiologyACR

The ACR encourages and supports nearly thirty-eight thousand radiologists, radiological oncologists, nuclear medicine physicians, and medical physicists in improving the practice of radiological care, the science behind radiology, and advancing the various radiological professions.

American Nurses Association (ANA)
8515 Georgia Avenue, Suite 400
Silver Spring, MD 20910
(800) 274-4262
Website: https://www.nursingworld.org
Facebook: @AmericanNursesAssociation
Twitter: @ANANursingWorld

The ANA is dedicated to supporting and advancing the nursing profession by establishing high standards and advocating for a safe and ethical workplace. The ANA also fights for issues relating to health care that affect nurses and the community.

American Registry of Radiologic Technologists (ARRT)
1255 Northland Drive
St. Paul, MN 55120
(651) 687-0048

FOR MORE INFORMATION | 71

Website: https://www.arrt.org
Facebook: @AmericanRegistryofRadiologicTechnologists
The ARRT provides technologists with licensing in medical imaging, radiation therapy, and various procedures of intervention by managing requirements in education, ethics, and exams.

American Society of Radiologic Technologists (ASRT)
15000 Central Avenue SE
Albuquerque, NM 87123-3909
(800) 444-2778
Website: https://www.asrt.org
Facebook: @MyASRT
Twitter: @ASRT
The ASRT is an organization that provides radiologic technologists with professional training and materials that can help them enhance patient care.

Bureau of Labor Statistics (BLS)
US Department of Labor
2 Massachusetts Avenue NE, Suite 2135
Washington, DC 20212-0001
(202) 691-5700
Website: https://www.bls.gov
This federal agency analyzes labor market activity, industry working conditions, and price changes in the US economy. Every year, the BLS updates the *Occupational Outlook Handbook* (https://www.bls.gov/ooh), which describes thousands of careers with details about job requirements and average salaries, including those in the radiology field.

Canadian Association of Radiologists
600–294 Albert Street
Ottawa, ON K1P 6E6
Canada
(613) 860-3111
Website: https://car.ca
Facebook and Twitter: @CARadiologists
The Canadian Association of Radiologists is the national professional organization dedicated to ensuring excellence in patient care and medical imaging among Canadian radiologists.

Commission on Accreditation of Allied Health Education Programs
25400 US Highway 19 North
Suite 158
Clearwater, FL 33763
(727) 210-2350
Website: https://www.caahep.org
Facebook: @CAAHEP
Twitter: @caahep
The Commission on Accreditation of Allied Health Education Programs reviews and accredits more than two thousand education programs in twenty-eight health care fields.

Health Canada
Address Locator 0900C2
Ottawa, ON K1A 0K9
Canada
(613) 957-2991

FOR MORE INFORMATION | 73

Website: https://www.canada.ca/en/health-canada.html
Facebook: @HealthyCdns, @HealthyFirstNationsandInuit
Twitter: @GovCanHealth
Health Canada is responsible for making sure that Canadians have access to the health services and care they need to reduce health risks and promote a higher quality of life.

Health eCareers
6465 South Greenwood Plaza Boulevard, Suite 400
Centennial, CO 80111
(888) 884-8242
Website: https://www.healthecareers.com
Facebook: @HealtheCareers
Twitter: @Healthecareers
Health eCareers is a website that provides information about job openings in the health care industry. The site also works to connect medical providers with qualified health care professionals.

FOR FURTHER READING

Agebagi, Steven S., and Elizabeth D. Agebagi. *Step-Up to Medicine* (Step-Up Series). 4th ed. Philadelphia, PA: Wolters Klewer Health, 2015.

Angulo, Roberto. *Getting Your First Job*. Hoboken, NJ: John Wiley & Sons, 2018.

Bushong, Stewart C. *Radiologic Science for Technologists: Physics, Biology, and Protection*. 11th ed. St. Louis, MO: Elsevier, 2017.

Fabbri, Christiane Nockels. *From Anesthesia to X-rays: Innovations and Discoveries That Changed Medicine Forever*. Santa Barbara, CA: Greenwood, 2017.

Hubbard, Rita L. *What Degree Do I Need to Pursue a Career in Health Care?* (Right Degree for Me). New York, NY: Rosen Publishing, 2015.

Leavitt, Amie Jane. *Jump-Starting a Career in Medical Technology* (Health Care Careers in 2 Years). New York, NY: Rosen Publishing, 2014.

Morkes, Andrew. *Hot Health Care Careers: 30 Occupations with Fast Growth and Many New Job Openings*. 2nd ed. Chicago, IL: College & Career Press, 2017.

Reeves, Diane Lindsey. *Health Sciences: Exploring Career Pathways*. Ann Arbor, MI: Cherry Lake Publishing, 2017.

Sheen, Barbara. *Careers in Health Care* (Exploring Careers). San Diego, CA: ReferencePoint Press, 2015.

Yate, Martin John. *Knock 'em Dead: The Ultimate Job Search Guide 2017*. Avon, MA: Adams Media, 2016.

BIBLIOGRAPHY

Allhealthcare. "Career Profile: Radiologic Technologist." Retrieved February 1, 2018. http://allhealthcare.monster.com/training/articles/242-career-profile-radiologic-technologist.

American Registry of Radiologic Technologists. "What Is ARRT Certification and Registration?" Retrieved January 19, 2018. https://www.arrt.org/about-the-profession/arrt-certification-and-registration.

BoardVitals. "Five Things to Know About the ARRT Radiography Exam." November 6, 2017. https://www.boardvitals.com/blog/about-the-arrt-radiography-exam.

Bureau of Labor Statistics. *Occupational Outlook Handbook*. January 30, 2018. https://www.bls.gov/ooh.

Burgess, Nancy. "What Is It Like to Work in Radiology?" Hospital Jobs Online. Retrieved January 12, 2018. https://www.hospitaljobsonline.com/career-center/healthcare-careers/what-is-it-like-to-work-in-radiology.html.

Carestream. "Q&A With Lead Radiologic Technologist at Scripps Health." March 21, 2012. https://www.carestream.com/blog/2012/03/21/qa-with-lead-radiologic-technologist-at-scripps-health.

Enelow, Wendy S., and Louise M. Kursmark. *Expert Resumes for Health Careers*. 2nd ed. Indianapolis, IN: Jist Works, 2010.

Fauber, Terri L. *Radiographic Imaging and Exposure*. St. Louis, MO: Elsevier, 2017.

Ferguson. *Exploring Health Care Careers*. 3rd ed. New York, NY: Ferguson, 2006.

Ferguson. *What Can I Do Now? Health Care*. New York, NY: Ferguson, 2007.

Field, Shelly. *Career Opportunities in Health Care*. 3rd ed. New York, NY: Checkmark Books, 2007.

Hayhurst, Chris. "The X-Files: The Past, Present, and Future of X-ray Equipment." *24x7*, June 8, 2015. http://www.24x7mag.com/2015/06/x-files-past-present-future-x-ray-equipment.

National Institute of Biomedical Imaging and Bioengineering. "Computed Tomography." Retrieved January 15, 2018. https://www.nibib.nih.gov/science-education/science-topics/computed-tomography-ct.

National Institute of Biomedical Imaging and Bioengineering. "Magnetic Resonance Imaging." Retrieved January 9, 2018. https://www.nibib.nih.gov/science-education/science-topics/magnetic-resonance-imaging-mri.

Quan, Kathy. *The Everything Guide to Careers in Health Care: Find the Job That's Right for You*. Avon, MA: Adams Media, 2007.

RadiologyEd.org. "The Radiology Career Guide." Retrieved January 22, 2018. http://radiologyed.org/careers.

Radiology Schools 411. "Advice for Getting Hired as a Radiologic Technologist." Retrieved January 24, 2018. https://www.radiologyschools411.com/careers/job-advice.

Wischnitzer, Saul, and Edith Wischnitzer. *Top 100 Health-Care Careers: Your Complete Guidebook to Training and Jobs in Allied Health, Nursing, Medicine, and More*. 3rd ed. Indianapolis, IN: Jist Works, 2011.

INDEX

A
American College of Radiology, 54
American Registry of Magnetic Resonance Imaging Technologists, 25
American Registry of Radiologic Technologists (ARRT), 28, 30, 36, 42, 43, 44, 45
artistic aspect, 64

B
Bureau of Labor Statistics (BLS), 17, 23, 28

C
camaraderie, 64
certification, 6, 24, 25, 30, 42, 43, 46
  exams, 6, 25, 28, 31, 42, 43
  preparation for, 43, 44–45
  strategies, 43
  programs, 24–25
communication skills, 33, 34
computerized tomography (CT) scans, 4, 14, 15, 17, 18, 21, 27, 28, 36
  certification, 65
  how they work, 14–15
constructive criticism, 37, 63
diagnostic information, 7

diagnostic medical sonographers, 16, 65
  education, 16
  income, 17
  job outlook, 16, 17
digital radiography, 14, 19

E
education, 5, 32, 37–39, 65
  associate's degree, 23
  community colleges, 5, 23, 32, 37, 39
  courses, 23, 32–33, 38, 39
  hospital programs, 5, 32, 34, 36–37, 39
  private institutions, 32
  universities, 37
  vocational school, 32, 37, 39
employment, 8, 18, 18, 37, 39, 40, 42, 51
  Advice for Getting Hired as a Radiologic Technologist, 37
  career path, 60, 65, 67
  rewarding experience, 4, 64
equipment, 4, 12
  evolution of, 12, 14
  specialized, 12, 21

F
film, 14, 19
flexibility, 10, 64

H

hands-on experience, 25, 34, 37, 39, 41

I

images, 4, 6, 7, 9, 14, 19, 22, 35
  3D, 15
  high-quality prints, 9, 20, 22, 38
  patient positioning for, 4, 9, 14, 27, 38
imaging devices, 6, 7, 9, 12, 22, 24, 40
  ionizing radiation, 12, 38
internships, 34, 39, 41–42, 54
  National Institutes of Health, 34
  pay, 41
  Rochester Institute of Technology, 34
  schedule, 41
  Southern Illinois Healthcare, 34
  success in, 41

J

job search, 46, 50
  applications, 49–50
  career centers, 50–51
  cover letters, 50
  interview process, 57, 59
  job fairs, 46, 51
  networking, 46, 54, 56–57, 67
  online postings, 46, 53, 54
  public libraries, 51, 53
  recruiters, 49, 50
  résumé, 46, 47, 48, 50, 51, 65
Johnson, Dennis, 26–27
Joint Review Committee on Education in Radiologic Technology, 24–25

M

magnetic resonance imaging (MRI) instruments, 15, 17, 18, 36
  how they work, 17
mammographers, 27–28, 65
  education, 27
  income, 28
  training, 27
mammography machines, 14
math, 23, 32, 33
medical ethics, 39
MRI technicians, 24, 25, 39, 65

P

patient interaction, 4, 7, 10, 18, 22, 25, 27
psychology, 23, 33

R

radiation, 11, 17, 18
  health department guidelines, 11
  protection against, 11–12, 18, 39

INDEX

safety, 11, 12
radiologists, 21, 28–29, 30, 32, 60, 65
  education, 21
  training, 21
radiology assistants, 28–31, 32, 60, 65
  certification, 30
  duties, 29–30
  education, 28, 30, 60
  patient interaction, 29
  training, 29
radiology department, 4, 8–9, 12, 21, 22, 28, 64
  hours, 9
radiology nurses, 31, 32, 65
  duties, 31
  education, 31
  NCLEX-RN, 31
Radiology Schools 411, 37, 39, 40, 56
radiology specialists, 21, 39
  demand for, 21
  traits, 34
radiology technicians, 4, 5, 6, 7, 9, 11, 18, 21, 22, 23, 24, 33, 34–35, 39, 40, 60
  demand for, 5, 23, 46
  desire to help others, 5, 6, 23, 34
  duties, 4, 11, 18–20, 22, 36
  education, 5, 21, 23, 28, 43

entry-level positions, 42–43, 61
importance to physicians, 4, 7, 9, 18, 64
income, 23
job outlook, 6, 23
licensure, 7, 21, 24
limitations, 11
rapport, 9
schedule, 4–5, 9–10
training, 4, 5, 7, 21, 24
workflow, 20
Roentgen, Wilhelm, 12, 14

science, 6, 23, 32–33
soft tissue, 7, 14, 16, 17, 24, 27

technology, 16–17, 23, 64

ultrasound technology, 16
  safety, 17
US Food and Drug Administration, 27

X-ray machines, 5, 7, 12, 14, 18
  how they work, 12–13, 14
X-rays, 4, 9, 11, 13, 14, 21, 38–39

About the Author

Jason Porterfield is a writer and journalist living in Chicago, Illinois. He has written many books for young adult readers, several of which have dealt with careers. These include *A Career as a Mobile App Developer*; *Careers as a Cyberterrorism Expert*; *Becoming a Quality Assurance Engineer*; and *Frequently Asked Questions about College and Career Training*.

Photo Credits

Cover (figure) Tatiana Gekman/Shutterstock.com; cover (background) Semnic/Shutterstock.com; back cover, p. 1 (background graphic) HunThomas/Shutterstock.com; pp. 4–5 (background) and interior pages Elnur/Shutterstock.com; p. 5 Pavel L Photo and Video/Shutterstock.com; p. 8 Alpa Prod/Shutterstock.com; p. 10 Skynesher/E+/Getty Images; p. 13 Science Source; p. 15 Du Cane Medical Imaging Ltd/Science Photo Library/Getty Images; p. 19 Tyler Olson/Shutterstock.com; p. 22 Klaus Tiedge/Blend Images/Getty Images; p. 24 Blend Images-Hill Street Studios/Brand X Pictures/Getty Images; p. 25 Kali9/E+/Getty Images; p. 29 Choja/E+/Getty Images; p. 30 Tempura/E+/Getty Images; p. 33 Hero Images/Getty Images; p. 35 Bill Bachmann/Science Source; p. 38 Medic Image/Universal Images Group/Getty Images; p. 44 Sidekick/E+/Getty Images; p. 47 John Moore/Getty Images; pp. 48–49 Simon Jarratt/Corbis/VCG/Getty Images; pp. 52–53 Bloomberg/Getty Images; p. 55 Klaus Vedfelt/Iconica/Getty Images; p. 58 Paul Burns/Corbis/Getty Images; p. 61 wavebreakmedia/Shutterstock.com; pp. 62–63 Jupiterimages/Creatas/Thinkstock; pp. 66–67 Ariel Skelley/DigitalVision/Getty Images.

Design: Michael Moy; Layout: Ellina Litmanovich; Senior Editor: Kathy Kuhtz Campbell; Photo Researcher: Sherri Jackson